DYING
CAN CHANGE YOUR
LIFE

To my wife.

Jeff Hastings
09/16/12

DYING
CAN CHANGE YOUR
LIFE

A Personal Testimony

of God's Grace

and Mercy

JEFF HASTINGS
WITH GWEN ELLIS

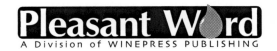

A Division of WINEPRESS PUBLISHING

Pleasant Word (a division of WinePress Publishing, PO Box 428, Enumclaw, WA 98022) functions only as book publisher. As such, the ultimate design, content, editorial accuracy, and views expressed or implied in this work are those of the author.

Unless otherwise noted, all Scriptures are taken from the Holy Bible, New International Version, Copyright © 1973, 1978, 1984 by the International Bible Society. Used by permission of Zondervan Publishing House. The "NIV" and "New International Version" trademarks are registered in the United States Patent and Trademark Office by International Bible Society.

Scripture references marked NKJV are taken from the New King James Version, © 1979, 1980, 1982 by Thomas Nelson, Inc., Publishers. Used by permission.

Scripture references marked KJV are taken from the Authorized King James Version of the Bible.

ISBN 13: 978-1-4141-0825-4
ISBN 10: 1-4141-0825-7
Library of Congress Catalog Card Number: 2006907199

TABLE OF CONTENTS

ACKNOWLEDGMENTS

My Mom who showed me what True Faith really is and led me along the path.

Mae Wood—Without your "motherly" prodding and encouragement, this book would have never been written.

Gwen Ellis—You sifted through my many files, listened and were on the "same page" with me.

To all the people I have known throughout my life, you each have taught me something.

And of course, God, there is who carried me through this journey.

Part I

MY STORY

You intended to harm me, but God intended it for good to accomplish what is now being done, the saving of many lives.

—Genesis 50:20

Chapter 1

WHEN YOU
HEAR THE WORST

My grace is sufficient for you, for My strength is made perfect in weakness.

—2 Corinthians 12:9 NKJV

It was 5:30 in the morning, and I was spilling coffee grounds all over. Great! Grounds in my coffee again! I was becoming an expert at keeping my teeth closed when I drank coffee.

I could make coffee in my sleep. So what was going on? It was the fourth or fifth morning in a row that this had happened. It was a simple, everyday task—take a scoopful of coffee and move it over to the coffee maker. Easy enough, but when I did that, the bottom of the scoop would hit the filter holder and coffee would go between the filter and the holder. Removing the filter and cleaning the grounds out of the holder was a skill that I was quickly perfecting.

The next morning, I was determined to not let it happen again. I concentrated carefully on scooping the coffee out of the can. I moved slowly, but then my hand began to shake as though I'd already had too much coffee. This had happened several times during the past few weeks. The slower I moved and the harder I tried, the more my hand would shake, until I just dumped the coffee into the filter. Sometimes I missed the filter completely. Now, as I stood looking down at my trembling hand and the scattered grounds on the countertop, other incidents surfaced that I had deliberately shoved to the back of my mind.

A few days before, a file folder that I was carrying at the office had slipped out of my hand, spilling the contents all over the floor. Similar incidents had happened several times in recent weeks. I'd shrugged them away in annoyance, giving the incidents no serious thought. Now I admitted to myself that for some time I'd had to make a conscious effort to keep from dropping things from my left hand. I'm left-handed, but I had instinctively started carrying file folders and books in my right hand.

It was also becoming increasingly hard to write. My handwriting was becoming smaller and smaller. And when I wrote, my hand would cramp up as if I'd just handwritten *War and Peace*. I was working for a major homebuilder at that time, and I had to sign 300 to 400 checks each month. This was becoming a problem.

As these thoughts flashed through my mind, I realized that this had been a gradual process over the last several months. Nothing dramatic—everybody drops things from time to time. Nobody's handwriting is 100 percent consistent all of the time. None of these things would have been significant as isolated incidents, but I realized they were happening more and more often. I could no longer deny that this was true, but I did try to rationalize it.

That spring, I had started playing softball. I hadn't played for 12 years. During practice, I noticed that my throwing arm was weak. I could barely throw a ball in from the outfield. When we had our first game, I played first base and experienced the same weakness. Twice I bounced the ball to the pitcher's mound. That experience convinced me that it was time to see my chiropractor. After a few treatments on my shoulder, the weakness in my arm was gone, and I quit worrying about it.

Now, it seemed logical to assume that my shoulder was acting up again. I would simply go to the chiropractor again, and he would straighten it out as he had done before. I also reasoned that these problems could be caused by stress. Stress can cause a lot of problems, and the past months had been very stressful for me. My mom had died a few months before in January 1999. I still missed her a lot. My dad was having serious heart problems. Or maybe this weakness was just me feeling my age. I didn't like that possibility. I was nearing 40, but surely that wasn't old enough to be having problems associated with old age. I decided to reject that idea.

It didn't occur to me that something could be seriously wrong. I'd had a physical a few months before and had checked out fine. So I decided to make a few visits to the chiropractor. I made an appointment immediately, but after a few sessions when there was no improvement, the chiropractor thought that my problem might be related to something neurological, and he referred me to my primary care doctor. Ironically, my chiropractor had buried his father-in-law the day of my last appointment, who had died from Lou Gehrig's disease (ALS), but he quickly dismissed that possibility because the disease attacks both sides of the body at the same time.

I went to see my primary care doctor. He was concerned, too, and sent me to a neurologist. The neurologist thought that I might be suffering from multiple sclerosis and made an appointment for me to have an MRI the following Saturday. I looked up MS on the Internet. What I found scared me to death. Multiple sclerosis is a cruel disease that recedes and then comes back, over and over.

I had the MRI on Saturday, and the following Monday I received a call from the doctor's nurse. She said that the doctor wanted to see me at my earliest convenience, even that day after work. I told her that it would have to be after work. She pushed me to tell her a convenient time—five o'clock? Six? Seven? I told her that I could be there by six o'clock. Her urgency alerted me that something was seriously wrong with me. Of course, everything that I'd read about multiple sclerosis flashed before my eyes. A doctor doesn't make a nighttime appointment to discuss an unimportant ache or pain. I tried not to imagine the worst, but I knew it was serious.

I called my wife and asked her to meet me at the doctor's office. When we got there, the doctor broke the news: I had a brain tumor. There's no way to soften such news, so he just told me this quietly. For a minute, I was actually relieved. My worst fear had been that I was suffering from MS, so I was relieved that it wasn't that. But then, slowly, the words sank in: brain tumor. Brain tumor = cancer = death.

Other than to tell us that more tests were needed and that we would later discuss the treatment, the doctor didn't give us a prognosis that night. He could see that we were in no condition to think clearly. When we left the doctor's office, my wife and I went to a restaurant on the Willamette River in downtown Portland, Oregon. We just looked at the river, held hands, and cried. The other people in the restaurant became a blur. We were hardly aware of them. I'm sure they knew something was wrong. Even though it was happy hour, we were anything but happy.

When we got home that night, my wife called her family and they gathered together at her mom's house. I didn't want to go. I don't know if I just didn't want to have to admit to others that I had a brain tumor—somehow talking about it would make it all the more real—or if I was afraid it would turn into a pity party. My wife dragged me there, and when I arrived, it was obvious they cared, even those I barely knew. My own family was 300 miles away, so it felt especially good to be with her family. I was glad I had come. My wife had known what I needed.

I felt that I was in a nightmare. I was numb, yet a thousand thoughts ran through my mind. Foremost was the realization that my life could soon be over. *So this is how my life is going to end. This is all I'm going to accomplish. This is it.* I kept thinking it couldn't be true. Surely this must be a horrible mistake. But I knew that it wasn't. I had a brain tumor—that was my reality now, and I could not escape it. A few days before I'd had it all. Life was good, and I thought that it would go on getting better and better. Then, with a few words from the doctor, the life as I had known it had ended.

I thought this was as bad as it could get. I was sure this was the worst moment of my life and that it couldn't get worse. But I was wrong. I didn't realize that night the full impact the tumor would have on my life. Nor did I realize that there would be other circumstances yet to be revealed that would also have devastating effects on my life.

We met with a neurosurgeon the following day. He scheduled me for a biopsy a few days later. The results of the tests showed that I had a malignant anaplastic astrocytoma tumor grade 3. Further tests determined that I had approximately three years to live. That was seven years ago. God had other plans for me, but I didn't know it at the time. In fact, I didn't know God very well at the time. I would, but that was still ahead.

That night, just hours after the diagnosis, I was filled with deep despair that allowed no hope of anything brighter to seep through. All I could foresee at that time was a short life filled with pain, hopelessness, helplessness, and fear for myself, my wife, and my children. What was going to happen to all of us?

The following promises from God weren't real to me at that time, but even so, God was fulfilling them (and many others) in my life. He gave me His strength and led me to Himself.

GOD'S PROMISES

And my God shall supply all your need according to His riches in glory by Christ Jesus.
—Philippians 4:19 NKJV

Blessed is the man who fears the LORD, *Who delights greatly in His commandments…He will not be afraid of evil tidings; His heart is steadfast, trusting in the* LORD.
—Psalm 112:1,7 NKJV

I lie down and sleep; I wake again, because the LORD *sustains me.*
—Psalm 3:5

It took awhile for this last assurance to become real to me. Even now, I can't say that I'm free from all fear, but I put those moments in God's hands, and He gives me peace. God's Word has proven to be true during the dark times of my life, and it sustains me at all times.

Chapter 2

CATCH ME WHEN I FALL

"For I know the plans I have for you," declares the Lord, *"plans to prosper you and not to harm you, plans to give you hope and a future."*

—Jeremiah 29:11

The main point that I want to get across in this book is that even though I wasn't always living for the Lord, He was always there to catch me when I was at my worst. My needs were always met—I was never homeless; I never starved. Although I struggled through the first years of my adult life, God always came through for me. No matter what was going on in my life, He made me aware of His presence. Philippians 1:6 says, *Being confident of this very thing, that he which hath begun a good work in you will perform it until the day of Jesus Christ* (KJV). That "good work" began the moment I accepted Christ. It became a part of my life because God made it so, not because I was living for Him.

My life up to this point had run a pretty normal course, with good times interspersed with some bumps and discouragements. I was born in Anchorage, Alaska, where my family and I lived for 15 years. I had a happy, normal childhood. My parents cared for one another and for their children. Their family came first.

As kids so often do, I took it all for granted. I knew that there was poverty and hardship in the world; I heard my parents talk about the war in Vietnam, and I saw it on the six o'clock news every night. My dad was a police officer during the years we lived in Anchorage, so I knew about crime and that there was a dark side of life for some people—but other people, not me. None of it really touched my life, nor did it ever occur to me that it would.

My biggest challenge as I grew up was my size. By the time I was 13, I was over six feet tall and still growing. I was shy and lacked self-confidence. Being tall and skinny during my teenage years became a real handicap to me. But there was nothing in my childhood years that would prepare me for the challenge I now confronted as I stood face to face with death itself.

My father was a strict disciplinarian. There were no gray areas with Dad—everything was black or white, truth or lie, right or wrong, yes or no. His rules were clear. His discipline was sometimes harsh, but always consistent. There were no negotiations and no peace talks with Dad. We knew what to expect if we disobeyed—swift, strong discipline. But his forgiveness was also swift.

When we did something wrong, Dad usually sent us to our room first to think about what we had done. There, we would wait for him to come and give us our punishment. Waiting was almost as bad as the punishment. Sending us to our rooms also gave him time to cool off, as my mom shared later with me. When it was over, it was over. I could get right back on his lap. There was no recrimination or browbeating. We were never made to feel ashamed or rejected.

I know now that God operates in the same way. We are told in Galatians 6:7 that *whatsoever a man soweth he shall also reap.* We are assured of His quick and full forgiveness when we repent: *Their sins and their iniquities will I remember no more* (Hebrews 8:10 NKJV).

Dad had no idea that he was following God's own pattern as he brought up his children. Following God's pattern wasn't one of his main concerns, but discipline and integrity were the basis of his character, and it was important to him that these virtues were taught to his sons. I think what kept me out of serious trouble during my teenage years—besides God's grace and mercy—was my desire not to disappoint my dad or mom. I respected my parents and wanted their pride and respect in return. I thank God for both of them.

While living in Anchorage, my mother attended a small Baptist church and took my brother and me with her. She accepted Christ and made a total commitment of her life to Him. When I was nine, I also accepted Christ as my savior and was baptized. I had a nine-year-old child's understanding of what Christ was about. I did not understand what it meant to commit my life to Him. However, in Hebrews 13:5, God assures us that He will never leave us nor forsake us. Now, as I look back, I realize that He has always been, and always will be, with me every step of the way.

Somehow, I knew that there was more to the Christian life than just walking down the aisle or being baptized. But I did nothing with my salvation during the years I was growing up. I don't think it was rebellion so much as it was passiveness. I have no explanation for that—I can't, and won't, claim the excuses I so often hear for people's lack of commitment.

My passiveness regarding my salvation certainly wasn't due to lack of example or training from my mother—she always lived her faith and tried to instill it in her sons. Nor was it because my dad didn't go to church or because of any lack in the teaching of my pastors or Sunday school teachers. I just accepted what Christ had done for me and gave nothing back. Even as a kid I realized this, but it would not be until my world fell apart in 1999 and I was forced to my knees in absolute helplessness and despair that I finally listened. My brain tumor didn't just happen; it took that event for God to bring me to Him.

When I graduated from high school in 1979, I took a year off to stay with my brother in Alaska and to work. I went to Washington State the following year to attend college at Central Washington University in Ellensburg. I went there for two years and did the typical college scene as far as partying, drinking, and so forth were concerned. Once in a while, I even studied at night. After my second year of college at Central, in the fall of 1982, I transferred to Washington State University (WSU) in Pullman. Everything changed for me at WSU. I didn't know anyone there, and I wasn't very good at making friends. To help with expenses, I took a job delivering newspapers in a rural area. I traveled over 100 miles per day on the route, six days a week—a lot of hours out of a school schedule.

I didn't learn very much at WSU. While I considered myself a fairly intelligent person, I didn't always demonstrate this fact. I started going to restaurants or bars nearly every night. I often drank heavily, which took a lot of money out of my tight school budget. One Thursday night, I became very intoxicated. Somehow, I managed to drive the few blocks to my apartment, where I continued drinking until I passed out. I woke up Friday morning sick as a dog. I'll spare you the grim details, but it was bad. All day long on Friday, I lay on the couch. I couldn't even stand up to get a drink of water or go to the bathroom without getting dizzy and sick.

The next day, Saturday, was also bad because I was so weak from lack of food and dehydration. I didn't know anybody, so I knew that no one would check on me. At times, I thought that I was going to die, because I couldn't get up. Knowing I'd done this to myself didn't help any.

As I lay on the couch that Saturday, I was aware of the presence of God. I lay there trying to pray, but the words wouldn't come. I tried to pray out loud and then I tried to pray silently, but regardless of what I did, I just couldn't get the words out of my mouth or out of my heart. I struggled, but nothing came out. Then Romans 8:26-27 came to my mind: *The Spirit also helpeth our infirmities; for we know not what we should pray for as we ought: but the Spirit itself maketh intercession for us with groanings which cannot be uttered. And He that searcheth the hearts knoweth what is the mind of the Spirit, because he maketh intercession for the saints according to the will of God* (KJV). At that moment, I gave it all to God and asked the Holy Spirit to pray for me. God gave me His peace.

That wasn't the last time I had to lean wholly on the mercy of God, even to the uttering of my prayers. But that Saturday morning, I had no inkling of what the future held for me. I was focused on the misery of the moment.

On Sunday morning, I woke up at 3:00 A.M. and felt pretty good. I had an overwhelming desire to be home in Wenatchee and in church. I left my apartment and got in my little Subaru four-wheel drive vehicle. The gas gauge was on empty when I started out, and it was snowing hard. The roads were slick with ice. This was definitely not the kind of weather to be out driving around in. But I knew the four-wheel drive vehicle would make it—if I could just find a gas station.

Because it was very early—before sun up—I couldn't find a gas station that was open in Pullman, Washington. But I knew that Moscow, Idaho, wasn't that far away, and it was the closest place I could think of where I might find fuel. I decided to take the chance that I had enough gas to make it to Moscow, eight miles due east of Pullman, but in the opposite direction that I needed to go. I had no other choice. At that point, I was absolutely determined to get to Wenatchee whatever it took. I finally did find a gas station, and soon I was back on the road.

During this time, the snow had not let up at all; if anything, it was coming down harder. It was still dark and the roads were icy. That strip of road was notorious for accidents even in the best of times, but I headed back to Pullman, got through town, and headed up the hill toward the west. The snow was so thick that I couldn't even see the top of the hill. But when I reached the top, I broke out of the storm and into beautiful clear blue sky and dry roads. It encouraged me so much, because I knew it was of God.

This experience has come to my memory again and again during the dark and fearful times that have come since that cold morning. It would later help me to understand that God's provision is always there through the dark valleys, and that the day will come when the sun will shine again. When we move into His light at the brow of the hill, we can look back into the valley and can say, "Oh, yes! All things do work together for good." Never doubt it.

In four hours or so, I got to Wenatchee. I walked into the church just as the service was starting, sneaked into the second row, and sat down. My mom, who was playing the piano, didn't see me. Everybody else did and, of course, they all knew me. I sat down by a Bible she had left in the pew (this was one of the Bibles that has brought me such comfort since her death). She played on, not knowing that I was there.

I'm sure everyone nearby was interested in seeing her reaction when she finally noticed me, and when it came, it was just as one would expect from Mom. As always, she was quiet in her reaction, but her smile and the brightness of her eyes said it all, loud and clear. She was surprised and glad to see me home and in church. But she was no happier to see me than I was to see her. I knew I was exactly where I was supposed to be.

I'm sure Mom knew that something was wrong, but we never talked about it. It wasn't her way to question. Praying was her way, not lecturing. She knew that I needed to be there with her. Her love was unconditional and obvious.

I never drank alcohol again. I don't know if I would classify myself as an alcoholic, but I do know that when I've had one or two drinks, all my will power disappears. This wasn't the first time I had become sick from drinking.

Usually, when people quit drinking, their old drinking buddies give them a bad time and they fall off the wagon. I don't know why but nobody did that to me. Actually, I do know why: God intervened.

You'd think that I would have learned my lesson after all that, but I hadn't. I was conscious of God, knew that He could see what I was doing, and never doubted Him. But I was not faithful to Him. His faithfulness to me during my unfaithfulness is beyond my understanding, but it is a clear testimony that He means what He says when He promised believers in Hebrews 13:5: *I will never leave thee, nor forsake thee* (KJV). He gave me nearly 20 more years to surrender my own self-will, but I refused. It was as if I were in a race to have as much fun as I could before God's wrath fell on me.

I think I was like the planter in the Parable of the Sowers (see Matthew 13:3-9). Some seed is planted on hard ground, and it doesn't take root at all. Some seed falls on rocky ground, and its root is so shallow it hardly grows. But then there is the other seed that falls on fertile ground. The roots go deep, and strong plants grow from this seed and bear fruit. God's Word fell on rocky ground in me. It took a long and painful time for that seed to root and grow.

God's Promises

Train up a child in the way he should go, and when he is old he will not depart from it.
—Proverbs 22:6 NKJV

But the Helper, the Holy Spirit, whom the Father will send in My Name, He will teach you all things, and bring to your remembrance all things that I said to you.
—John 14:26 NKJV

Call to me and I will answer you and tell you great and unsearchable things you do not know.

—Jeremiah 33:3

Chapter 3

GAINS AND LOSSES

*Who is he that overcometh the world, but he that believeth
that Jesus is the Son of God?*

—1 John 5:5 KJV

S oon after my trip to Wenatchee, I dropped out of
college. During the next two years, I worked both
in Alaska and Wenatchee. By 1987, I was again living full-time in Wenatchee, and I started working in real
estate. In 1989, I went to work as Operations consultant
at the headquarters in Salt Lake City, and after a year, in
1990, I moved to Vancouver, Washington. While working for this company, I met the woman who became my
wife.

We were married in 1990 and I became an instant
father. She had three small children from a previous
marriage. Our daughter, Ashley, was born the following
year—a year in which I gained a daughter but lost another
job. The company I was working for went out of business.

We moved back to Wenatchee, and I got another job in real estate. At first that job sounded good, but no sooner had we arrived in Wenatchee than there were changes within the company and my new job evaporated.

I went from one great opportunity to another great opportunity, only to see them all fizzle out. My going from job to job never allowed us to get settled. Each month, our finances became more and more of a struggle.

In 1994, our son Adam was born, but this time when I gained another child, I also got a good job. I went to work for one of the biggest builders in the Vancouver area. Six months later, that company went bankrupt. Now I was getting a complex—and I was also becoming very concerned.

I was supporting a family of seven, and it was a huge struggle to care for our needs. However, in 1995 I went to work for another builder, and life improved considerably. I worked there for three-and-a-half years, and then in July of 1998, a major housing developer hired me. This was the most lucrative and promising job I'd ever had. It was my dream job. The future suddenly looked much brighter.

I was excited to have an opportunity to work for this well-known company. I found satisfaction in my position as manager. I liked my coworkers and supervisor; it was exactly the kind of work and atmosphere I had been hoping for. For the first time in my career, I felt that I had obtained security and stability.

Shortly after I went to work at this company, my wife was also hired at the same firm. Our multiple family schedules were working out fine. Adam, who was just past four, went into daycare, and the other kids were in school during the day. I was sure that our family had turned a corner in our lives and that we were now on a new and firm foundation.

My own personal integrity and work ethic had always prompted me to put my best effort into every job I'd ever had, but this job was especially important to me. I studied every phase of my responsibilities and learned all I could about the company. I worked long hours and found satisfaction in every moment of it. Of course, all this meant that I went home very tired and had little time or energy for my family. I regret that. It wasn't that my job was more important than my family, but I knew that how I did my work determined my success or failure on the job and that it would have a direct and long-term effect on the welfare of my wife and children. There is no way to achieve success without hard work and long hours, and it was finally paying off. I took it for granted that my wife understood and shared my goals.

I remember so well one particular afternoon when I came home from work and sat in my car in the driveway thinking about my life. I was 38, I had a great job that brought me a sense of satisfaction and accomplishment, a good marriage (or so I thought), five wonderful kids, and I had just signed a contract to build a beautiful new home—a big change from the uncertainty of the previous years. We were young and healthy. The future was bright. Life was good.

I don't know why I didn't see the cracks developing in the foundation of our marriage. I guess my rose-colored glasses blocked out the growing clouds on the horizon. Or perhaps I subconsciously blinded myself to the danger signals, preferring to focus on seeing my dreams come true. It was such a relief to have something other than uncertainty and worry to think about.

I used to wonder if there was anything I could have done to prevent the breakup of my marriage. But actually, I doubt it. In any case, that kind of thinking is useless and nonproductive speculation. Then Mom died on January 13, 1999. Even now, those stark words—Mom died—have the power to bring sorrow. For a while, that grief pushed all else from our minds.

Ironically, just the month before, my dad had a routine MRI, and the doctors had found an aneurysm that required immediate surgery. Because of the seriousness of the operation and the possibility he would not survive, Dad went to the funeral home a few days before the surgery was scheduled and made arrangements for his own funeral and cremation. He had wanted to save Mom the stress of having to make these arrangements. However, the careful plans that he made were destined to be used for her.

Mom had a bad cough at the time and found it easier to sleep sitting up in her lounger rather than lying in bed. So Dad had decided to sit up with her. Years before,

INTRODUCTION: Job

Suffering is a test of trusting
God for who He is and
not for what He is allowing
to happen

in 1973, she had a pacemaker installed, and then had a stroke in 1986, but other than the cough, she seemed to be doing pretty well. Then during the night (which happened to be the 25th, anniversary of her mother's death) Mom died quietly in her sleep. On the day Dad would have been having surgery, we instead had a memorial service for Mom. Dad had surgery a few days later and lived another two years.

A short time after Mom's death, I found this note written in her own handwriting on the page before the book of Job in her Bible. The writing was childlike. She had to learn to write again after a stroke. The note said."

Suffering is a test of trusting God for who He is
And not for what He is allowing to happen.

Many times over the past years, I have found handwritten notes, old prayer lists, and comments in her Bibles. They are a source of encouragement to me now, just as her presence was when she was alive.

Even though Mom had been ill for a long time, her death was a tremendous shock. No matter what was going on in my life, she had represented love, strength, stability, and even refuge. But I also know that when Mom died, I did not lose her. I know exactly where she is: In a better place.

The kids and I had talked with her on the phone the night before her death. Adam told her, "Grandma, I know what your phone number is: 1-800-COLLECT." Knowing my mom, I'm sure she shared that little comment with my dad. I can imagine them laughing together. Just hours later, she was dead. I could hardly comprehend that I could no longer pick up the phone to hear her voice. There was a definite and painful void in my life.

I had always had a premonition that something bad was going to happen to me. This feeling was probably a natural result of my subconscious awareness that I was not living as God would have me live. When Mom died, I thought that the premonition of something bad about to happen had been fulfilled. Her death certainly was something bad happening to me. But there was more to come—much more.

I no longer believe that God took Mom to punish me, but I do believe He used her death to get my attention. It did make me think about eternity and my own mortality, but I still didn't yield my life to Him—I kept putting it off, planning to do it later. I was young, and I had years to take care of that—or so I thought. We all think this when we're young.

My wife had always had a real affection and respect for my mother. She grieved her loss along with the kids and me. We all missed Mom. I think Mom's death slowed the deterioration of our marriage, but it didn't prevent the inevitable. I could no longer deny that we both wanted to separate. Even so, we stayed together, with neither of us making that first move toward divorce. We lived separate lives in the same house, seldom seeing each other, and not really knowing how to communicate with one another. Tension grew greater by the day.

The fact that I didn't react quickly and strongly to save our marriage was probably an indication that my own love and commitment had been deteriorating along with hers, and because I didn't want to break Mom's heart. I was becoming more and more accepting of the fact that divorce would be our next move, and I even began to think of it as a way out of what had become an intolerable situation.

Oddly, considering everything else, we did start visiting various churches in our community, but we never went more than two or three times to any one church. I believe this might have been a time when we could have turned things around if we had actually brought God into our lives, but we didn't. And that failure brought its own consequences.

In Ephesians 5:22-23, Paul instructs wives to submit to their husbands, but he also includes a passage after that for husbands. All too often, we stop short of this Scripture: *Husbands, love your wives, just as Christ also loved the church and gave Himself for her...so husbands ought to love their wives as their own bodies* (vv. 25,28). Perhaps if husbands underlined this verse in their Bibles, read it every day, and asked God to enable them to do this, more marriages would be saved. But I didn't do that, and so what happened next was inevitable.

GOD'S PROMISES

It is written: "Eye hath not seen, nor ear heard, neither have entered into the heart of man, the things which God hath prepared for them that love him.

—1 Corinthians 2:9 KJV

But those who hope in the Lord will renew their strength. They will soar on wings like eagles; they will run and not grow weary, they will walk and not be faint.

—Isaiah 40:31

And we know that in all things God works for the good of those who love him, who have been called according to his purpose.

—Romans 8:28

Chapter 4

TROUBLE IN PARADISE

Do not let your hearts be troubled. Trust in God; trust also in me.

—John 14:1

By February 1999, our lives were pretty much back to what passed for normal for us—two people living under the same roof, not fighting, not yelling, not name calling, but just exhibiting total indifference toward each other, leading their own separate lives. Nothing had changed in our marriage, but it was about this time that I first began to notice physical changes in myself. For instance, as I mentioned previously, my left hand would relax, and without warning I would drop whatever I was holding. Once in a while, I would stumble a little, and my writing was erratic. These incidents were not frequent and were over in seconds, easily dismissed until the next time they occurred.

A major part of my job was to know everything that was going on in the various housing development projects from Southwest Washington to Northwest Oregon—what progress was being made, what problems or potential problems were happening, which architectural designs were being used, and so forth. I had a good memory, so it was easy for me to remember even the small details. But suddenly, I began to find myself struggling to answer a question that ordinarily I could have answered at once, or searching for a name or a word I knew well.

Memory loss was harder to dismiss than physical symptoms, but still these episodes didn't happen all that often. It was annoying, but not alarming. What an amazing capacity we have for deliberately deceiving ourselves! Not until I started playing softball and had so much trouble throwing the ball did anything really catch my attention and prompt me to seek help. Even then, I didn't connect my shoulder problem with the other problems that I was experiencing in my life.

As I mentioned, I went to a chiropractor, and after a few visits my shoulder seemed fine again. Once again, I shoved it all aside. If a nagging worry did slip into my thoughts, I reminded myself that I'd had a physical not too long before and that I had been pronounced fit and healthy. I rationalized that whatever was wrong couldn't be all that serious.

However, by late spring when I began to spill coffee every time I tried to make a pot, I had to recognize that there was definitely something wrong. The outcome of all the ensuing doctors' visits and tests was undeniable and irrevocable. My life was twisted beyond recognition. An inoperable brain tumor was my reality. Everything else faded. I saw my future as a dark tunnel of pain, radiation, chemo, eventual disability, and death. I would not see my children grow up. I would have no future success in the business world, no big bank account, and certainly no reconciliation in my marriage. This hopeless picture was firmly planted in my mind. As time passed, God would change that hopelessness to hope and peace, but at the time of the diagnosis, I felt nothing but terror and anger that this catastrophe was happening to me.

My wife stood beside me. This wasn't reconciliation, and neither of us thought that it was. But I will never forget her willingness to put aside her personal plans to help me. And I did need her help and encouragement. For the next few weeks after the initial diagnosis, we put our differences aside and focused on my treatments. We even let our original plans to move into our new house go forward, mostly for the sake of the children.

Shortly after my tumor was diagnosed in August 1999, she and I met with the radiologist to discuss the treatment plan, which was very detailed. In September, the radiation treatments began and continued through October. A mesh mask was made to hold my head still so that the radiation would hit my tumor only, not the rest of my head. That was a weird feeling. They laid a piece of warm, wet string mesh over my head and then shaped it to my face. My eyes, nose, and mouth were covered. I thought

I was going to suffocate. It seemed like forever before it hardened, but it was actually only a few minutes.

Then the technicians cut eyeholes and nose and mouth holes. A template—a four-inch thick piece of lead—protected the rest of my brain from being exposed to radiation. The beam was computerized so that it would only go so deep and hit the same spot each time. Thank God for the medical knowledge we now have.

These treatments lasted six-and-a-half weeks. Five days a week at 8:00 A.M., the technicians strapped that mask on me as I lay down on the radiation machine. The treatment itself lasted about 20 minutes. For the first few radiation treatments, I drove myself to the appointment after I dropped the kids off to school and daycare. I preferred it that way. I didn't want to deal with anyone's pity. Occasionally, it was necessary to take the younger children with me. They sat in the waiting room and watched TV.

The first two weeks weren't too bad. I thought, *This is going to be a piece of cake.* But as time went on, the radiation began to have an effect on my body. I started getting tired more often. I'd usually take a nap as soon as I got home from treatment. I didn't get sick, just weaker and weaker.

One morning, about three weeks into my radiation treatments, my hair started falling out in the shower. At first, it was just a few hairs. As the days went by, I had two bald spots above my ears. The next weekend we went to visit my dad and brother and everyone took a turn shaving my head. There was an odd aspect to this. Over the previous years, once in a while I would have a weird dream in which I was standing in a shower and my hair was falling out. I wasn't vain about my hair and I didn't have the dream often, just once in a while, but now that dream was coming true.

During one of the meetings with the radiologist, my wife asked the doctor how long she thought I had to live. The doctor told us that the median survival rate was three years, which meant that if 100 people have a brain tumor, 50 of them would die within three years. My wife broke into tears. I didn't ask about the other 50 people. Many factors go into the mix, including a person's basic health and the current treatment. My dad believed that a positive attitude had a lot to do with healing. He recognized and encouraged this attitude in me, and I think it encouraged him as well. I hope Dad realized where I found my positive attitude—in God.

After the radiation was finished, I took a break in my treatment. On my birthday in November, my wife took me on a surprise visit to Seattle, Washington. It was cold, and the wind was blowing so hard that it seemed to cut right through my jeans. I was freezing. So she went to the store to buy me a pair of sweats. She was gone longer than I thought she should be, and I started to worry, as it was growing dark in downtown Seattle. Then I saw her coming down the street. As we hurried to the ferry, I was very glad to have those warm clothes.

We went to a bed and breakfast in Bainbridge Island that my wife had rented. The bedroom looked across

Puget Sound to the west side of Seattle. It was very beautiful. I had never seen Seattle from this viewpoint.

In December, I began to notice that my entire left side did not want to work. However, the corporation I was working was having their annual Christmas party in San Francisco, so I decided since I had finished radiation and had not yet started chemo, I would go to the party and wait to see the oncologist until I got back. When I returned, the doctor put me on a steroid to reduce the swelling in my brain that was causing the numbness in my left side. I gained 45 pounds in two-and-a-half months, which was obvious even on my six-foot-five frame. Gradually the swelling went down, the numbness went away, and I was left with maybe 50 percent capacity on my left side. It affected my coordination, and I had to learn to write with my right hand.

Another challenge I faced was reading. It was tough for the first year or so for me to read. I couldn't seem to concentrate long enough to understand what I was reading. I couldn't focus my eyes or keep my place on the lines. I would be reading and all of a sudden realize that I was daydreaming. Most of the time, I would read for about five minutes and then fall asleep. Gradually, though, as time passed, my reading time increased, and my naptime decreased. At the time, I even had trouble comprehending or following along in the Bible. Now, I read several chapters in the Bible each day.

I learned very quickly that when you are first diagnosed with a life-threatening condition, "friends" come out of the woodwork with all kinds of stories of miracle cures. They bombard you with articles (all lacking details or any way to verify them) that they say will be the answer to your prayers. These people all mean well. They are only trying to be helpful and encouraging. But it's like a tidal wave washing over you. You wait and wait for that miracle in a bottle to wash up on the bank and save you from the nightmare, but it doesn't happen. Eventually, the tidal wave of "helpers" recedes and never comes back. Except for the most weird of them, there is deafening silence. But there was one exception for me.

One special doctor who cared for me during my illness deserves special recognition—a Chinese doctor named Dr. Joe. A friend of my wife referred us to Dr. Joe. My wife made an appointment for me without my knowing it. I had already made the decision that I wasn't going to use any crackpot cures, so when she told me about this Chinese doctor, I was reluctant. But to pacify her, I went along with her plan.

When we went to Dr. Joe's office, all along one wall of the office we saw plastic jars of different herbs and roots. The combination of smells was stifling at first, but we quickly got used to it. We sat for a while, nervously staring at each other. The office was in a small house, and we were in a back room. Don't get me wrong—the room was light and clean and everything was professional. It was just plain and different from any doctor's office I had been in before.

Then in walked Dr. Joe, with a smile on his face. His whole demeanor was very calming, and he was soft spoken. He shook my hand, held on to it and said, as if he were reading my mind, "Know this, there is no magic pill to cure cancer. If anyone tells you they have one, turn around and run." I liked him immediately.

Dr. Joe then turned my hand over and put his hand on my wrist as if he was checking my pulse, but it was more than that. I'm not going to say he was reading my mind, but I was later to find out that he could accurately tell people's moods.

My left side had become increasingly numb and paralyzed. After talking for a while with Dr. Joe, he said he wanted to do acupuncture on me. He explained that once the swelling went down in my brain, the use of my left side would come back, and the acupuncture would keep the nerve paths connected. Nobody had told me about my being a pincushion, but I agreed to go along with the procedure.

I'm not a doctor (and I don't play one on TV), but it made sense to me. Acupuncture didn't hurt. It kind of tingled. As I lay there, Dr. Joe would poke holes in my skin with needles and I'd feel a little tingle run up my leg or arm. I liked this sensation, because it was the only feeling I had in my left side. And it felt good.

I had the acupuncture treatments two or three times a week. Dr. Joe also prescribed a mixture of herbs. These were mainly to counteract the effects of the radiation and chemo and to keep my blood levels up, not to cure me. He boiled a mixture of herbs in a tea or broth and put them in individual plastic pouches. I don't know what was in the mixtures, as he wrote the ingredients in Chinese.

I drank one of these each night before I went to sleep. It tasted terrible—as bad as sweaty feet smell! I'd pour it into a cup and set it on my nightstand, crank up my will power, and then gulp it down as fast as possible. Then I would quickly lie back and hope and pray that stayed down. Drinking these mixtures became easier as time went on. As far as the acupuncture went, I knew that I would have to wait to find out how effective the treatments were. It wasn't helping the numbness on my left side, but Dr. Joe hadn't expected it to—it was just supposed to maintain the nerve connections.

As time went by, I got to the point where I could hardly tie my shoes or button my shirt (not to mention my pants). I came close one day to having to ask one of my coworkers to help me zip up my pants in the men's room at work, but somehow I managed to do it. At one appointment with Dr. Joe, he ended up tying my shoes because he couldn't bear to watch me struggle with the laces.

I had a hard time walking. I was constantly dragging my foot or missing steps. This was mostly due to the swelling in my brain. I could also barely move my fingers. Writing was out of the question. I couldn't even hold a pen in my left hand—and I'm left handed! Even as I'm writing this book, I'm alternating between writing with my left hand and my right hand.

I don't know how much the herbs helped, but they surely didn't hurt me. And I do know that Dr. Joe's understanding and compassion was good medicine.

We were still not moved into our house by Christmas day 1999, but we decided to take the kids to see their new home. We put a big red ribbon on the front door and hung a huge red Christmas stocking inside from the stair rail of the second floor. We showed the kids through the house and explained to them that it was our family Christmas present. They were thrilled with all the bedrooms and the large finished daylight basement that would be their recreation room. It was big enough for them to play in, and they could bring their friends.

I can't describe my reaction as I watched the children running through the house. I knew it was all an illusion. I asked myself what in the world I was doing in letting my marriage continue. I wondered if I would even be alive by next Christmas—and if I were, what condition would I be in? Would we still live here in this new house? What was going to happen to my children when I was gone?

I knew, of course, that in the event of my death or total incapacity, their mother would have to do it all. She would have responsibility for all five of them, two of whom were special-needs children. I felt guilty for leaving her by dying and wondered if she could really handle all of it. I was helpless to control these thoughts and the resulting frustration. I was also helpless to find the answers.

Now, I look back on that time from the perspective of what God has done for me, the peace of mind He has given, His provision of all our needs, and the assurance that He will always care for my children. But right then, before I had yielded my life completely to Him, I viewed everything through the distortion of despair.

We moved into our new home on December 30 and, for a little while, for the sake of the children (and the season, too, I suppose), My wife and I continued to maintain the facade of a happy family. But we knew that in reality, we were living a lie. A home built on the sands of a crumbled marriage and terminal illness will not stand—and ours didn't.

GOD'S PROMISES

Trust in the Lord with all your heart and lean not on your own understanding; in all your ways acknowledge him, and he will make your paths straight.
—Proverbs 3:5

I will lift up my eyes to the hills—From whence comes my help? My help comes from the LORD, Who made heaven and earth.
—Psalm 121:1-2 NKJV

Be joyful in hope, patient in affliction, faithful in prayer.
—Romans 12:12

Chapter 5

GOING OUR OWN WAY

What shall we then say to these things? If God be for us, who can be against us?...We are more than conquerors through him that loved us.

—Romans 8:31,37 KJV

The year 2000 started quietly enough. The dire predictions of Y2K did not materialize. However, for my wife and me, our lives would quickly yield to their own upheaval. The facade we'd built around ourselves for the past few months began to deteriorate.

My life was pretty much out of my control for several months. The radiation treatments were over, but now the chemotherapy would begin. In addition, a decision had to be made about my work. I was still employed, but I hadn't been very productive, and that was not going to change for some time to come, if ever. I knew my time of employment was over for the foreseeable future. However,

I didn't expect the blow that hit me when I went into the office the first week of January.

Through a set of circumstances that took me totally by surprise and over which I had no control, my honesty and integrity at work came into question. I had no defense for the accusations presented against me without exposing the person responsible for making the change, and I was not willing to do that. Of all of the agonizing things I had endured and faced, this black mark against my character was the most difficult to bear. Cancer might eventually destroy my body, but that paled in the face of this accusation that hit at the heart and soul of who I was.

Even during the years I was away from God and all through the weaknesses of my college years, integrity was always a priority for me. I would never have knowingly committed an act of dishonesty to the degree I was being charged. If I could have chosen between my keeping my character or my health, I would have chosen my character. But I lost both. I literally could not have borne that loss without God's sustaining strength.

I wish I could say that the issue was resolved and my innocence proven, but even today it is still unresolved. Nor will I say that I understand why God allowed this to happen or that it no longer pains me. It does, but I can say with peace and honesty that I trust God in this matter. I trust His promise in Romans 8:28; that all things work together for our good when we trust Him. And I trust His declaration in Malachi 3:6: *I am the LORD, I change not* (KJV). He will take care of it. A friend brought this quotation from Oswald Chambers' book *My Utmost for His Highest* to my attention: "Neither a lie or the truth will be hidden forever." I can trust and rest in that promise.

My wife and I discussed our situation, and we agreed that it would be best if she moved in with her mother and stepfather. The kids would stay with me. This may sound daunting under the circumstances, but the house was large and there was room for all five kids to keep on with their lives and schedules without undue interruption. They were all in school during the day, and when they were home, they seemed to sense that I needed their support. It worked out quite well. However, I knew that this would only be a temporary arrangement and that it was imperative I face reality. I was determined that the son and daughter that my wife and I had in our marriage would stay with me, and I had to make provisions for them. In the ensuing divorce action, my wife and I were granted joint custody, but she generously allowed Adam and Ashley to live with me.

I was feeling better, but I still had the chemo treatments ahead. They were to begin immediately in a series of six-week cycles that would continue for a year. Between these chemo treatments (which left me very weak), having to deal with public agencies regarding Social Security, Medicaid, HUD housing, and the myriad of other decisions I had to make, I suffered some serious blows to my pride.

I had never been judgmental or had any feeling of superiority to people who needed help, but the experience of having to deal with the public agencies did increase my compassion and understanding of others. I learned, first hand, how quickly and unavoidably you can find yourself cashing a public assistance check instead of a paycheck. I learned about waiting rooms and waiting lists. I learned about answering the most personal and invasive questions and about completing forms and applications that left me feeling worthless and nonproductive. I learned about helplessness. I felt that I no longer had control of my life.

I had been praying and submitting my circumstances to God, but finally I got on my knees and put everything in His hands—including my children, who are dearer to me than my own life could ever be—and openly accepted whatever He had for me, be it a long life or short one.

In July 2000, I ended a chemo cycle. I now had six weeks of freedom until I had to start another cycle. My dad had asked me to bring the kids and come stay with him during the summer break, so Ashley, Adam, and I went to Wenatchee to spend the next six weeks with him. My wife moved back into the house with her other three children.

Dad was still living in the home that he and Mom had shared. It was a good time for all of us—there was a wonderful swimming pool in the backyard, and my brother lived nearby, as did three of my mother's sisters, and numerous cousins. Ashley and Adam spent most of their time in the pool, and we had family picnics and backyard barbeques. I think it was an especially good time for Dad. Even though it had been more than a year since Mom's death, he still missed her a lot, and the kids seemed to give him a new interest. I am especially glad today that we had that time with him. He died a few months later on March 18, 2001.

When the kids and I returned to Vancouver, my wife and I decided that she and the other three children would stay in the house while Ashley, Adam, and I found other housing. Neither of us had any desire to reconcile by this time. I didn't have the energy to try to make our marriage work. What was the point?

My wife told me later that she felt guilty of "abandoning me," but I didn't feel that way. We were caught in an impossible situation, and regardless how it had come about, it could not be changed. It was useless to blame anyone—there is nothing more futile or destructive than the blame game. I just no longer cared, nor did I care what anyone else thought about the situation. This is not to say that it didn't hurt to lose my marriage. It did. It just hurt less than struggling to make it work. For a while, we called it a "trial separation," but we knew that our marriage was over. Ultimately, we filed for divorce.

I was now faced with the dilemma of how I was going to survive. I started going to church, and I committed my life to God. I asked that He make the rest of my life productive for Him, and that is what has happened, is happening, and will continue to happen. My life is and will continue to be a testimony to Him and will bring glory to His name. Everything I have is in His hands—all of it, including my children. It's the best place to be, because there is no greater security for them or for me. May His will be done. God soon began opening doors. He brought little miracles. He reminded me of His promise that if I obeyed Him, He would provide for me. And He did.

While I was not technically homeless, I didn't have any place to go. My wife's mother and stepfather asked me and Ashley and Adam to move in with them. It was an answer to prayer, and I appreciated it more than I can ever express. They generously opened their home to the man who would soon be their ex-son-in-law and to two active children aged six and nine. That was quite a change for two people who were used to having their home to themselves.

Another blessing came after I applied to the local Housing Authority for rent assistance. I was approved, but I was put on a waiting list and told that the usual waiting time was two years. That could be a lifetime for me. As generous as my in-laws had been, I don't think they had a two-year time period in mind when they asked us to live with them! Fortunately for me, the Housing Authority put me on their "terminal" list. The Housing Authority estimated that the time I would have to wait to receive a house on that list would be about six months. Basically, I would be waiting for someone to die. I felt like a vulture.

Two months from the time I first applied, I got a call from someone at the Housing Authority telling me that my name was now at the top of the list. All I had to do was to find housing that qualified, and they would pay a portion of the rent.

There were apartments up the hill from my in-laws that were fairly new. The grounds were very nice and, best of all, the complex was family-oriented. There was a large pool and playground for the kids. In fact, I had often thought that if I had to live in an apartment, that's the kind of place I'd like to live. I asked the lady at the Housing Authority if the apartments in that complex were approved. She said they were. The apartment manager also approved, and we got a ground floor apartment that opened into the courtyard with the play area. It was perfect. God knew exactly what we needed, and He provided.

At the same time, my disability supplement came through. It was a provision straight from God. In February 2001, we moved into the new apartment. However, we lacked furnishings. The kids had their beds, but that was all the furniture we had. Then my dad called and told me he wanted me to be comfortable, so he told me to pick out a bed and a recliner. The Lord led me to find unbelievable deals. I started realizing more and more that God was working in my life. My faith was growing.

Once again, things were leveling off and I was beginning to relax a little when another blow struck. On March 18, 2001, I got another call. It was from my brother, Andy. Dad had died.

To my knowledge, my dad never accepted Christ as his Savior. This added to the grief I felt at his death, but then I remembered that he had taken Mom to church for two years after her stroke in 1986 when she couldn't drive and that he had stayed with her during the service. I don't know whether my mom and dad are together now. He had heard the Word and knew the plan of salvation. Dad did have the opportunity to accept Christ. My brother also found one of Mom's Bibles opened on Dad's nightstand after his death. Only my dad could have put it there. My hope is that Dad did make a decision for Christ. I only regret that I didn't express more to Dad about the peace God was giving me during my illness.

Just as Dad had an opportunity to make his decision, I had one to make now.

I had one of two ways to go as I dealt with this fresh grief. I could rail at God, or I could choose to trust Him. Again, the litany of my disasters ran through my mind. In less than two years I had lost both my parents, my own life was in jeopardy, and I'd lost my career, home, marriage, and reputation. Would it ever end? As clear as anything could be, I knew I was at a crossroads. I could continue to trust God, or I could hold on to the catastrophes of the past two years and turn my back on Him. Faith or bitterness—the choice was mine.

I made a choice for faith, although I didn't understand all that had happened to me. But then, that's the real test of faith—trusting God and His never-changing promises even when the circumstances of life seem to contradict everything we believe.

Soon the pieces began to fall into place and a picture began to form. I gradually came to realize that it had taken the brain tumor to bring me to God in complete faith and submission. Now, I can thank God for that tumor. I'd rather be as I am now, in the security of God's protection and care, than in the security of anything this life can offer. I thank God for doing what He had to do to bring me to Him.

GOD'S PROMISES

One of the two which heard John [the Baptist] speak, and followed Him, was Andrew, Simon Peter's brother. He first findeth his own brother Simon, and saith unto him, We have found the Messiah, which is, being interpreted, the Christ.

—John 1:40-41 KJV

Seek ye first the kingdom of God, and his righteousness; and all these things shall be added unto you.

—Matthew 6:33 KJV

Ask and it will be given to you; seek and you will find; knock and the door will be opened to you.

—Matthew 7:7

Chapter 6

GETTING TO KNOW GOD

Humble yourselves, therefore, under God's mighty hand, that he may lift you up in due time. Cast all your anxiety on him because he cares for you.
                                        —1 Peter 5:6-7

I knew I would die sometime; we all know that. *Sometime* being the operative word—*sometime* when I was so old I wouldn't care anyway; *sometime* in the dim and distant future, when my great-grandchildren were standing at my knee or sitting on my lap, not my own little boy and girl. However, in my situation, *sometime* had come; *sometime* was now. In a moment of time, at the age of 39, I was standing face-to-face with death.

Hearing the medical prognosis that I probably had, at the most, three more years to live straightened out my priorities really quickly. Although I'd been a Christian for 30 years, I had never yielded my life to Him. That realization had actually never been completely out of mind, but now it was right up front.

At the time, I wasn't thinking that I would experience a miraculous New Testament healing. I didn't fall to my knees and start begging God for healing or try to make a bargain with Him in exchange for a longer life. It didn't occur to me to seek out a healer, but very quickly, what I had learned as a child in my home and in the churches we had attended came back to my memory. I didn't consciously remember when I'd learned or been taught the Scriptures that I now found myself reading or remembering, but it was clearly the Holy Spirit leading me to God's Word. God never fails to keep His promises.

I went to several churches. My former pastor's son was pastoring a church a mile from my home in Vancouver, but the thought of going to a church with ties to my past did not seem to fit right at this point. I didn't want to go there. I was afraid I would feel too much pressure and obligation to attend. So I attended larger churches, where I could easily slip in without being noticed. No one knew me, and I knew no one there. I admit that I made little effort to get to know anyone. I just sat near the back and left as soon as the service was over. It was an empty feeling.

Finally, I went to my former pastor's son's church. It felt like my old church in Alaska. It felt like home. I knew the doctrines of the church were sound and fundamental. I didn't have to worry about learning or evaluating new things. I could relax in the friendly atmosphere and concentrate on strengthening my renewed relationship with God. After attending a few weeks, I went forward and publicly rededicated my life to God. A flood of emotion came over me. It had been a long time since I had felt such peace.

I knew that, with God's help, I would have to face my fears regarding my condition. So after the children left for school each day, I began to spend the better part of the mornings studying God's Word and praying for His guidance and peace. I found great strength in Psalm 56:3-4: *When I am afraid, I will trust in you. In God, whose word I praise, in God I trust; I will not be afraid. What can mortal man do to me?* In fact, what could man do to me?

It is so weird when you finally break through and realize that this world is not what's important. When there is nothing left but God, that's when you find out God is all you need. I thought back over the years and tried to trace the beginning of my first awareness of God's presence and the realization that I needed to make a commitment of my life to Him. I knew that I had always been aware of Him, but I think God really got hold of my thoughts after Mom died, even before I received the diagnosis of my brain tumor. I had started looking through one of the several Bibles Mom had and compared her Bibles to mine.

My Bible was 20 years old, but it was just like new. Not a mark or a wrinkle marred it. However, in Mom's Bibles, verses were marked and highlighted throughout. There were notes in the margins, and I found old prayer lists, some that were 20 years old. Little pages from *Our Daily*

Bread were torn out and stuck in the pages of her Bible. Her faith and love for God were genuine. I read over and over again the scriptures she had specifically marked, and I began to realize even more fully her love and concern for her sons. But it wasn't until after my diagnosis, radiation, and chemo treatments, and the full realization of my prognosis that I got down to business myself.

I remember one morning in particular when a note left in one of Mom's Bibles provided an especially inspiring moment for me. Ashley and Adam had just left for school. I poured myself a fresh mug of coffee and started my daily reading. That morning I was reading in Proverbs. I noticed a speck near one of the verses and tried to brush it away. It wouldn't come off. I looked at it more closely and realized it was a pen mark. It was by Proverbs 1:11, and there was another mark by verse 15. Each verse began "My son...." The verses weren't underlined, but nevertheless, it was a deliberate mark to call attention to them.

I was reminded of Hebrews 11:4: Though she is dead, yet she speaks. Mom couldn't have left a greater legacy.

Because Mom obviously got a lot of strength from the book of Job, I bought a study guide on that book. I knew a little bit about Job, but I didn't know he suffered so much. I had heard about the "patience of Job," but that's all I really knew about him. Actually, I don't see the patience of Job in the book that bears his name. What I see is his perseverance and his faith. He had some moments of discouragement and anger, but through it all, he held to his trust in God and emerged from suffering into blessing and restoration. During Job's life, God doubled everything that he'd lost. And through it all, God protected his soul—which is what we should be worried about anyway. That's what is important.

I don't know why, but it was more than a year before I could look at pictures of Mom, especially to look her in the eyes. It hurt too much, and perhaps I was ashamed. In addition, I was the only one in the family who didn't dream about Mom for a long time. My only contact with her was through her Bibles. Somehow, I think, she asked God for that.

With the diagnosis of an anaplastic astrocytoma grade three tumor in my brain, I embarked on what has been a fascinating and exciting life journey. It hasn't been easy, nor do I expect it to be. There were, and are, moments of fear and despair. This tumor was God's provision for awakening within me my need of Him every moment—an awareness I wouldn't have had if my life were centered on usual problems and responsibilities. That's what I want to share with you.

For to me to live is Christ, and to die is gain (Philippians 1:21 KJV). This is an easy verse to quote, but a hard one to live by. It's just not as simple as that. We can quote it all we want, but when death hits us square in the face, the words fade. Wanting to give up the gift of life that God Himself created and granted us is not natural to us, nor should it be. But as we read the Bible and grow in our relationship and understanding, the principle becomes clearer.

In Mark 10, there is an account of Jesus healing a blind man. I'd heard and read that story since I was a kid, but I had not realized the personal application for my life. Finally, I did. Jesus stopped and said, *Call him* (v. 49). So they called to the blind man. Notice the blind man's response: *Throwing his cloak aside, he jumped to his feet and came to Jesus* (v. 50). Immediately, Jesus told him, *Go…your faith has healed you* (v. 52). In these few words we find the key to every provision and promise in the Bible: faith and obedience.

When I finally heard God's personal message for me in these simple words, I knew that He was calling me out of a different kind of blindness. I realized that He had been calling me since I answered His promise of salvation at age nine, but that I had ignored His voice and stumbled on in my own willful blindness, always knowing there was something more but refusing to let Him open my eyes. But this is my testimony now:

> *Before I was afflicted I went astray, but now I obey your word… It was good for me to be afflicted so that I might learn your decrees.*
>
> —Psalm 119:67,71

Looking back on my situation, I believe that the greatest gift God that gave me is that *I have no baggage!* I don't dwell on things. Not only did God guide me through my illness, but he also reached down and dug me out of the mess of the worldly system—the rat race that I was involved in. I have no animosity for those who hurt me, whether they did so intentionally or not. In fact, I feel sorry for some of them. And I don't hate the friends who abandoned me.

I have a clear conscience about everything in my past because it led me here—to this moment. I don't think God had this in mind when He created me, but He used my circumstances to bring me back into fellowship with Him. And there is no place else that I'd rather be.

GOD'S PROMISES

For God did not give us a spirit of timidity, but a spirit of power, of love and of self-discipline.

—2 Timothy 1:7

Jesus answered and said unto them, Verily I say unto you, If ye have faith, and doubt not, ye shall not only do this which is done to the fig tree, but also if ye shall say unto this mountain, Be thou removed, and be thou cast into the sea; it shall be done.

—Matthew 21:21 KJV

Therefore we do not lose heart. Though outwardly we are wasting away, yet inwardly we are being renewed day by day.

—2 Corinthians 4:16

Part II

WHAT I HAVE LEARNED

Two things I ask of you, O Lord; Do not refuse me before I die:

Keep falsehood and lies far from me; give me neither poverty nor riches, but give me only my daily bread.

Otherwise, I may have too much and disown you and say, "Who is the Lord?" Or I may become poor and steal, and so dishonor the name of my God.
                                              —Proverbs 30:7-9

Chapter 7

PRAISE GOD FOR THE HAMMER, THE FILE, AND THE FURNACE

I counsel you to buy from me gold refined in the fire, so you can become rich; and white clothes to wear, so you can cover your shameful nakedness; and salve to put on your eyes, so you can see.

—Revelation 3:18

A group of Bible students were studying Malachi when they came upon a verse they did not understand: *He will sit as a refiner and purifier of silver; he will purify the Levites and refine them like gold and silver. Then the LORD will have men who will bring offerings in righteousness* (Malachi 3:3). Why would a refiner of silver have to sit beside the refining vessel? Just what is the process for refining gold and silver? One of the students decided to find out the answer to these questions by visiting a silversmith to see the refining process in action.

As the student watched, the silversmith first took a piece of silver and held it with tongs over the center of the fire. The silversmith explained to the student that when refining silver, it is necessary to hold the piece of silver over the hottest part of the fire, as this burns away all the impurities. The silver is then melted into a molten mass.

The student asked the refiner if he truly needed to sit by the molten metal the entire time. Couldn't he go off and attend to some other duties and then return at a future time to find the silver refined? The silversmith assured the student that he needed to sit and watch the metal the entire time, for if the silver was left too long in the fire, it would be destroyed.

After watching the process and thinking for a few minutes, the student asked the refiner how he would know when the silver was pure. The silversmith replied that was the easy part—it was when he could see his face in the molten metal.

The agony of a man's affliction is often necessary to put him into the right mood to face the fundamental things of life.

—Oswald Chambers

Why does it take an earth-shaking event to make us stop and evaluate what is important in life? Why does one have to be thrown in the crucible of fire to figure out that God is trying to get our attention? Why did I have to have a catastrophic illness to understand that God loved me and was calling me?

I was a lot like Jonah before my illness. God wanted me to go in one direction, but I had my own ideas. I had a plan for my life and went my own way until I ran into an obstacle that I couldn't work around, climb over, or walk away from. An inoperable brain tumor is not something you can ignore. My tumor was like Jonah's whale. It swallowed me up and consumed my life—and brought me to my senses.

When I was diagnosed with having an inoperable brain tumor, God suddenly had my attention. I was 38 at the time and found myself in a helpless situation that neither I nor any doctor could change. The stress in my life became unbearable. It was like a cauldron of fire. I prayed for calm, but it never came. Instead, the stress grew until it twisted every facet of my life. In a matter of weeks, I literally lost everything except my children. And I didn't have a clue how I was going to care for them.

But like the refiner sitting and watching over the melting silver, God was watching over me. He knew how much it would take to get my full attention. I had turned away from God, but He had never turned away from me. He loved me and wanted me to come back to Him.

It just isn't in God's nature to abandon his children. So, while God didn't create my troubles, He certainly used them to bring me back to Himself. Today, I can honestly say that I wouldn't give up what He has given me since my diagnosis for anything I might have achieved in my life if I had been allowed to move along a more normal course.

Eventually, I lost it all: my job, my wife, my parents, my health, and my house. But what I lost was material, physical, and temporal. What I gained was eternal: peace, grace, trust, and the love of God. When you put what I've lost side by side with what I've gained, there's no comparison. I won! And I know that the best is yet to come.

Praise God for the Hammer, the File and the Furnace. The Hammer molds us, The File sharpens us, And the Fire tempers us.

—Samuel Rutherford

Each of us has been and still is being refined by the Master Refiner. What are some of the qualities of silver and gold that he'd like to bring out in us? Let's examine a few of these qualities.

First, both silver and gold reflect light. Silver is used as a film coating on the back of mirrors to reflect an image. Gold, when polished to a high finish, will also reflect light with a warm glow. However, neither gold nor silver have an internal light of their own—they are like the moon in that they can only reflect the light of the sun. In the same way, we can only reflect the light of God's Son. The more pure we are, the more refined we are and the better we will be able to reflect His light and glory.

Gold and silver are also beautiful. Since the beginning of history, these two metals have been treasured by all cultures. Think of the gold and silver treasures of the Pharaohs or those of the Aztecs and Incas. Of course, before gold and silver can become items of beauty, they have to be cut and fashioned by a craftsman. Ultimately, the beauty of the adornment will be determined by the tooling that is done on the piece. The more intricate the design, the more beautiful the piece. In the same way, God will often tool us through various difficult circumstances that come our way so He can fashion us into items of great beauty and worth.

Gold and silver are excellent conductors of both sound and electricity. Silver has a pure acoustic ring and is often used for bells and musical instruments. Compact discs pressed on 24-karat gold provide the ultimate in sound quality. Gold circuitry was used in the Pathfinder's robotic geologist to transmit information back to Earth from Mars and is used in computers to relay information from the keyboard to the microprocessor. In fact, gold is essential in computer circuitry because of its electrical conductivity and lack of degradability over time. In the same way, God wants each of us to be conductors—conductors of His love and grace. However, just as gold and silver must first be refined before they can be used as conductors, God first must refine our lives before He can use us for His glory.

Silver can be refined in a certain way for use as a purifying agent. For many years, silver was used to kill bacteria. Silver nitrate drops were used to clean the eyes of newborns, and silver solutions are still used today in the treatment of burns. Silver chemically affects the cell membranes of bacteria, causing them to break down, and the bacteria do not develop resistance to silver as they do to many antibiotics. During my experience, God showed me that one of our primary functions as Christians is to purify the environment around us by introducing others to Christ, speaking up for truth and righteousness, and by living a life above reproach. Yet, like silver, before we can be used as a purifying agent, God may first have to refine us through adversity.

Gold is used to protect. In fact, gold is used to protect the President whenever he flies on Air Force One. The metal can confuse an incoming missile's heat-seeking signal so that its guidance system cannot focus on its target. In the same way, God will use us to protect others. Christians who live in this world serve as a deterrent to evil. Because we live here on Earth and are filled with God's spirit, we hold back the forces of evil.

Thank God for the Trials

All of us must choose the path
We'll take for our life,
Some are narrow, some are rough
And some look smooth and wide.
The bright sunshine, it comes and goes,
The air is clean and warm.
And other days the dark clouds bring a thunderstorm...
Yet in any situation I have learned to be content.
For through the rain, a rainbow He has sent!

Thank God for the trials
That help make us strong,
Thank God for the music
His merciful songs,
Thank God for a savior
Who carries us along,
Thank God for the trials
That help make us strong.

—Laura A. Lohmeyer
Copyright © 1998

In the end, just as gold and silver that has passed through the refining process become beautiful and useful, so we, when we are passed through the Refiner's fire, become beautiful in God's sight. We become useful to Him. It is a process that God has been using to refine individuals for thousands of years. In fact, we find it happening again and again throughout Scripture.

Consider the adversity that Joseph endured. He was sold into slavery by his brothers, imprisoned for a crime he didn't commit, and forgotten by those who promised to help him. Yet through it all, God had a plan for Joseph's life. He used the evil that his brothers and others did to refine him into a great leader who would one day save a nation. In the end, Joseph could stand before his brothers and say: *You intended to harm me, but God intended it for good to accomplish what is now being done, the saving of many lives. So then, don't be afraid. I will provide for you and your children* (Genesis 50:20-21). God has a plan for our lives and will work everything that happens to us for our good.

The prophet Samuel anointed David to be the next king of Israel. However, before this could occur, David had to go through a series of trials. King Saul, who was jealous of David's successes in battle, relentlessly hunted David down. On several occasions, David had to flee the land and hide up in the hills just to save his life. He must have felt neglected and abandoned by God and fearful for his very life. Yet he proclaimed:

> *The Lord is my shepherd, I shall not be in want.*
> *He makes me lie down in green pastures,*
> *he leads me beside quiet waters,*
> *he restores my soul.*
> *He guides me in paths of righteousness*
> *for his name's sake.*
> *Even though I walk*
> *through the valley of the shadow of death,*
> *I will fear no evil,*
> *for you are with me;*
> *your rod and your staff,*
> *they comfort me.*
>
> *You prepare a table before me*
> *in the presence of my enemies.*
> *You anoint my head with oil;*
> *My cup overflows.*
> *Surely goodness and love will follow me*

> *all the days of my life,*
> *and I will dwell in the house of the Lord*
> *forever.*
> —Psalm 23:1-6

Even when we walk through the valley of death, we don't have to fear evil, for God is with us. God is there whenever we call on Him. But first, we must call.

Perhaps the greatest example of one who was refined by the fire was Job. Job was a wealthy man with land, status, possessions, and many children. Yet God allowed the devil to test Job and take away everything he had. A group of marauders came through and carried off his oxen and donkeys, killing his servants. Fire fell from the sky and burned up his sheep and other servants. Raiding parties swept down and carried off his camels, and killed more of his servants. His sons and daughters, who were feasting in a home, were killed when a mighty wind swept in and toppled the structure.

Yet despite these trials, Job proclaimed, *"Naked I came from my mother's womb, and naked I will depart. The Lord gave the Lord has taken away; may the name of the Lord be praised"* (Job 1:21). Job realized that God had given him everything he had and that He had the right to take it back, whether he was a good steward of those resources or not. Even when Job himself was afflicted with painful sores that covered his entire body, he refused to curse God. In the end, Job realized, *Those who suffer he delivers in their suffering; he speaks to them in their affliction* (Job 36:15).

So if you, dear friend, find yourself in the midst of impossible circumstances, take heart. Listen for the voice of God. You will find that He is calling to you and that He wants to draw you to Himself. God can use everything that happens to you to His glory, if you will allow it. If you feel as if you've been thrown into the midst of a fiery furnace, know that God is with you.

Also remember that sometimes God is the Refiner, looking on, but at other times He is actually *in* the fire with you. Think of the three Hebrew children in the book of Daniel: Shadrach, Meshach, and Abednego. King Nebuchadnezzar tossed them in a furnace that had been heated seven times hotter than normal. And what happened? When those in attendance looked into the furnace, they saw a fourth figure walking around with them in the fire. Amazingly, the only thing that had burned was their bonds. The fire had set them free! The observers said that it appeared that the fourth person was "a son of the gods." They were partially right—it was not a son of the gods, it was *the* Son of God. Sometimes God looks on, but sometimes He walks through the fire with us.

If you are in the fire, realize that God is near. He is watching you. He loves you and is concerned for your wellbeing. And He knows what He is doing. At the end of the refining process, you will come forth as pure gold.

Throughout my illness, and even today, God's Word has been an encouragement to my heart. Here are some Scriptures that have blessed my soul when passing through the fire.

GOD'S PROMISES

*But he knows the way that I take; when he has tested me,
I will come forth as gold.*

—Job 23:10

*The refining pot is for silver and the furnace for gold, But
the LORD tests the hearts.*

—Proverbs 17:3 NKJV

*I will refine them like silver and test them like gold. They
will call on my name and I will answer them; I will say,
"They are my people," and they will say, "The LORD is
our God."*

—Zechariah 13:9

*"He redeemed my soul from going down to the pit, and I
will live to enjoy the light." "God does all these things to a
man—twice, even three times—to turn back his soul from
the pit, that the light of life may shine on him."*

—Job 33:28-30

Chapter 8

PATIENCE IS MORE THAN A VIRTUE

*Our soul waits for the L*ORD*; He is our help and our shield.*
For our heart shall rejoice in Him, because we have trusted
in His holy name.

—Psalm 33:20-21 NKJV

The proverb "patience is a virtue" has been traced back to a book called *Piers Plowman*, written in A.D. 1377 by William Langland (the proverb is similar to the Latin *maxima enim patientia virtus*, "patience is the greatest virtue," and the French *patience est une grant vertu*, "patience is a great value"). The need for patience has not decreased in the hundreds of years that have passed since Langland first coined the phrase. When I was diagnosed with a malignant brain tumor, I entered the "school of patience and waiting." I found myself waiting in doctor's offices and hospitals. I waited for test results. I waited and hoped for good news. It seemed as if I was always waiting for the next step, the next something, the next...I knew not what.

I was not alone in the school of waiting. Most of us have at one time or another encountered situations in our lives about which we can do little except wait. That puts us in the same category as most of the great heroes of the Bible.

When we read the Bible, it often seems as if one miracle followed right on the heels of another. We see the great victories of the Bible warriors as happening one after another. But the truth is that sometimes hundreds of years passed between the miraculous events that we read about in the Word of God.

Think about it. Noah waited 100 years for rain as he blindly followed God's command to build the ark. It wasn't until he finished the craft that the rain came in abundance. Abraham and Sarah waited decades for a son after God had promised Abraham that his seed would be as the sands of earth and the stars of the heavens. After it was humanly impossible for the couple to become parents, God gave them the promised son. Joseph waited many years for vindication after his brothers sold him into slavery. It wasn't until many years later—when his brothers appeared before him begging for his help—that he knew his waiting was over and he revealed his identity to them.

When Joseph was about to die, he told the Children of Israel that God would lead them to the land that He promised to Abraham. He said, *God will surely come to your aid, and then you must carry my bones up from this place* (Genesis 50:25). Yet the Children of Israel would have to wait 400 years until God delivered them from bondage in Egypt. Probably neither Joseph nor any other person alive to hear his request dreamed that it would be 400 years before the exodus would occur.

After God called Moses to lead the Children of Israel out of Egypt, they had to wander 40 years in the wilderness before they could enter the Promised Land. Granted, their wandering was because of their sinfulness and stubbornness, but they still had to wait to enter into the rest that God had promised them.

The whole nation of Israel—and indeed the world—then waited for a Redeemer, a Messiah, to come. When Mary, a young woman from the small town of Nazareth, learned from an angel of the Lord that she would give birth to God's Son, the waiting was almost over. Jesus was born into the world and eventually paid the ultimate price for our sins through His death on the cross.

Today, believers wait for the return of that same Messiah to take us home to be with Him forever. Psalm 130:6 says, *My soul waits for the Lord more than watchmen wait for the morning.* There is no patience without the waiting—it's part of the process. We ask God for what we need (or what we think we need), and then we wait.

I Asked God

I asked for strength that I might achieve;
I was made weak that I might learn humbly to obey...

I asked for health that I might do greater things;
I was given infirmity that I might do better things...

I asked for riches that I might be happy;
I was given poverty that I might be wise.

I asked for power that I might have the praise of men;
I was given weakness that I might feel the need of God...

I asked for all things that I might enjoy life;
I was given life that I might enjoy all things...

I got nothing that I asked for—but everything I had hoped
for;
Almost despite myself, my unspoken prayers were
answered.

I am among all men most richly blessed.
                                        —Unknown Soldier

Charles Stanley, a great preacher of our time, once said, "Stop praying for a lighter cross, and start praying for strength to bear it!" That's the way it is. Tough times will come to all of us, and we must wait with patience for God to move. One of the most important lessons that I've learned from suffering with a brain tumor is that there are many situations that we simply can do nothing about. We have to have patience and wait and trust God. We have to depend on God to move in our tough situations. There is no other way.

After being diagnosed with an inoperable brain tumor, I tried to start a support group, but I was getting stalled every time. I couldn't get anyone to help and I could find no place to meet. I prayed and prayed about it, but nothing happened. When I talked with others, they immediately saw problems instead of offering solutions. So I continued to wait and pray about the situation.

Finally, I stepped out in faith and set up a meeting, even though I still had no place to hold it. And wouldn't you know it? God blessed us with two places to hold the meeting—we had to make a choice between the two! It's just like God to provide more than we asked, better than we asked, and exactly when we needed it. Patience coupled with prayer brought the answer.

Because of my lack of energy, I have had to learn patience. Up until my illness began, I was able to do just about anything that I made up my mind to do. But now, when I am busy doing something physical, I will all of a sudden feel very tired. I've learned to ask God for energy, and He gives it—but gradually, not immediately. In fact, often I am working when all of a sudden I realize that energy has come to me so gradually that I didn't even notice.

I'm still learning to ask God for little things, such as getting the kids up, taking care of their safety and mine, asking Him to give me an appetite, and even requesting His help to increase my memory and focus. I'm still learning to thank and praise Him for the joy, peace, faith, hope, strength, and courage that He provides.

Speaking of patience, God certainly had patience with me as I wandered my way through life. I know without a doubt that I became a Christian at the age of nine. But then I got in with the wrong crowd and drifted away from God. I went to church until I was 18, and then finally stopped going altogether. But in spite of not going to church, I still believed in God. Then I found out that I had a brain tumor, and with that diagnosis came the knowledge that God has always been there to watch over me—to catch me when I fall. Somehow, in my darkest times when the light shone through, I knew it was God.

It's interesting that during those very difficult days when I lost my job because of my illness, I didn't ask God for anything. I didn't have the guts to ask. Yet in spite of my reluctance, God didn't let me or my family starve. He provided for our needs. I was able to receive Medicare for the kids and me. We were able to have adequate housing that God provided through the Housing Authority. God gently and patiently wooed me back to Himself with His provision, love, and kindness. He is an awesome God! I don't know how much time God will give me here on Earth, but I do know that I want to serve God every day that I have left.

There is a wonderful story in the Old Testament about Hagar, a slave girl in Abraham's household, who became the mother of Abraham's child. As we mentioned, God had promised that He would bless Abraham and his wife, Sarah (or Sarai, as she was then known), with a son. However, after many years of waiting, Sarah worried that she was getting too old to have children. So she came up with the idea of having her husband make a baby with Hagar. Shortly after Hagar became pregnant, Sarah grew jealous and was so hard on Hagar that the girl fled into the desert. But God was watching. He knew exactly what Sarah had done to Hagar, and He came to talk with Hagar about it:

> The angel of the LORD found Hagar near a spring in the desert; it was the spring that is beside the road to Shur. And he said, "Hagar, servant of Sarai, where have you come from, and where are you going?"

> "I'm running away from my mistress Sarai," she answered.

> Then the angel of the LORD told her, "Go back to your mistress and submit to her." The angel added, "I will so increase your descendants that they will be too numerous to count."

> The angel of the LORD also said to her: "You are now with child and you will have a son. You shall name him Ishmael, for the LORD has heard of your misery. He will be a wild donkey of a man; his hand will be against everyone and

everyone's hand against him, and he will live in hostility toward all his brothers."

Genesis 16:7-12

The next part is the one that has such meaning for those of us who are patiently waiting for God: *She gave this name to the LORD who spoke to her: "You are the God who sees me," for she said, "I have now seen the One who sees me"* (v.13).

Oh, to see the One who sees us! That is great joy! That is the place where peace happens in our life. That is the place where we no longer have to fake trust and faith, for we know His love and promises are true.

If you are in a waiting place, take heart. God sees you. He is near. He loves you. He wants you to relax in your circumstance and trust Him. So look for the One who sees you. Lean back into His love and let it enfold you.

GOD'S PROMISES

Wait for the LORD; be strong and take heart and wait for the Lord.

—Psalm 27:14

For in thee, O LORD, do I hope: thou wilt hear, O Lord my God.

—Psalm 38:15 KJV

Never will I leave you; never will I forsake you.

—Hebrews 13:5

Chapter 9

EXPERIENCING GOD'S MERCY

Let us then approach the throne of grace with confidence,
so that we may receive mercy and find grace to help us in
our time of need.

—Hebrews 4:16

There once was a man named George Thomas, a pastor in a small New England town. One Easter Sunday morning, he came to the church carrying a rusty, bent old birdcage. He set it by the pulpit.

Eyebrows in the congregation were raised. As if in response, Pastor Thomas then began to speak. "I was walking through town yesterday," he said, "when I saw a young boy walking along and swinging this bird cage. On the bottom of the cage were three little wild birds, shivering with cold and fright. I stopped the lad and asked, 'What you got there, son?'

'Just some old birds,' he replied.

'What are you gonna do with them?' I asked.

'Take 'em home and have fun with 'em,' he answered. 'I'm gonna tease 'em and pull out their feathers to make 'em fight. I'm gonna have a real good time.'

'But you'll get tired of those birds sooner or later,' I said. 'Then what will you do?'

'Oh, I got some cats,' said the little boy. 'They like birds. I'll take 'em to the cats.' I was silent for a moment. Then I asked the boy, 'How much do you want for those birds, son?'

'Huh?' he replied. 'Why, you don't want them birds, mister. They're just plain old field birds. They don't sing. They ain't even pretty!'

'How much?' I asked again. The boy sized me up as if I were crazy and said, '10 dollars.' I reached in my pocket and took out a 10-dollar bill. I placed it in the boy's hand. In a flash, he was gone. I then picked up the cage and gently carried it to the end of the alley where there was a tree and a grassy spot. Setting the cage down, I opened the door, and by softly tapping the bars persuaded the birds to come out, setting them free."

Well, that explained the empty birdcage on the pulpit to the congregation. And it is a perfect picture to us of God's mercy. Those little birds were captives of a cruel master, but then they were purchased by someone who had mercy. The pastor didn't have to spend the money. He didn't really have any good reason to do so besides the fact that he wanted to extend a hand of mercy. And so he not only bought the birds, but he also set them free.

Mercy is
God *not* giving
you what you *deserve*.

Grace is
God giving you
what you *don't deserve*.

I was kind of like those birds in a cage. I was trapped by my own reluctance to follow God closely. I was headed in the wrong direction. God used my brain tumor to get my attention and bring me close to Himself. Although it might not have seemed like it at the time, that was an act of mercy. Then God showed even more mercy to me and extended my life well beyond the time the doctors thought I would live. That has been mercy not only to me but also to my children as well.

There are so many times in the Bible when God could have (and probably should have) wiped the human race off the face of the Earth. Think of the story of the Great Flood as told in the book of Genesis. Yes, the punishment God handed out to the planet was severe, but He showed mercy to Noah, his family, and the species on the Earth by saving them from destruction.

Think about all the times that God set out to destroy the Israelites, who were prone to wander in their affections toward Him. And think of how He often relented and showed mercy to them because of His great love for them. One of those times is recorded in the book of Numbers.

After God led the Israelites out of Egypt, the people grew impatient with wandering in the desert and lacking the food with which they had become accustomed. Many of them voiced their bitterness to God and to Moses. Well, the Lord soon had enough of their complaining and sent poisonous snakes to bite and kill them all. Many of the people died before those still living admitted that they had sinned when they spoke against God and against Moses.

Although God was angry at the Israelites, He had mercy on them. When Moses prayed for the people, God told him to make a bronze snake and put it on a pole. Moses followed God's command, and anyone who had been bitten by a snake and who looked at the pole experienced God's mercy and lived (see Numbers 21:6-9).

> *When they discover*
> *the center of the universe,*
> *a lot of people will be disappointed*
> *to discover they are not it.*
> —Bernard Bailey

There's an interesting story about a group of scientists who decided that humans could do without God. One of them looked up to God and said, "We've decided that we no longer need You. We have enough wisdom to clone people and do many miraculous things." God listened patiently and then said, "Very well, let's have a man-making contest. We'll do it just like I did back in the old days with Adam." The scientists agreed, and one of them bent down and picked up a handful of dirt. God looked at him and said, "No! You have to make your *own* dirt!"

Like the Israelites, we often think that we know what is best for our lives. We cry out in our circumstances and complain that God is leading us into suffering. We want to go back to the land of Egypt, where at least we had some sense of security. We worry that God has forgotten His promises and try to force His hand through our own actions. We forget that God is the *sovereign Lord* and that He has the right to do anything He wishes with us—and in His own time.

Fortunately, in His mercy, God has patience with us. Like a loving parent, He corrects us and guides us down the paths He wants us to take. He created us, He loves us, and He died for us. He doesn't owe us anything. But each time we lock ourselves into the cage that our sins create—each time we presume that we don't need Him—He reaches into our lives with His forgiveness, unlocks the cage door, and sets us free.

There is a wonderful old poem called "The Hound of Heaven" that tells how God pursues us until we give in to His love. A portion of this poem reads like this:

I fled Him, down the nights and down the days;
I fled Him, down the arches of the years;
I fled Him, down the labyrinthine ways
Of my own mind; and in the mist of tears
I hid from Him, and under running laughter.
Up vistaed hopes I sped;

And shot, precipitated,
Adown Titanic glooms of chasmèd fears,
From those strong Feet that followed, followed after.
But with unhurrying chase,
And unperturbèd pace,
Deliberate speed, majestic instancy,
They beat—and a voice beat
More instant than the Feet—
"All things betray thee, who betrayest Me."

God comes looking for us, and in His mercy He pursues us until we fall into His love. Here are the closing lines of the poem:

"Rise, clasp My hand, and come!"
Halts by me that footfall:
Is my gloom, after all,
Shade of His hand, outstretched caressingly?
"Ah, fondest, blindest, weakest,
I am He Whom thou seekest!
Thou dravest love from thee, who dravest me."

God's love often leads us down roads where earthly comforts fail us. Paul said, *To you it has been granted on behalf of Christ, not only to believe in Him, but also to suffer for His sake* (Philippians 1:29 NKJV). When we come to the end of all our dark valleys, we'll understand that every circumstance has been allowed for our ultimate good. As Bible teacher F.B. Meyer once said, "No other route would have been as safe and as certain as the one by which we came. If only we could see the path as God has always seen it, we would have selected it as well."

God's love and mercy are truly limitless. That's what caused Him to send His only Son to die in our place. Our God cares that we come into fellowship with Him. He cares that we are wayward and trapped in a cage of our own sinful making. He wants to set us free.

There's a Wideness in God's Mercy

There's a wideness in God's mercy
like the wideness of the sea;
there's a kindness in his justice,
which is more than liberty.
There is welcome for the sinner,
and more graces for the good;
there is mercy with the Savior;
there is healing in his blood.

There is no place where earth's sorrows
are more felt than in heaven;
there is no place where earth's failings
have such kind judgment given.
There is plentiful redemption
in the blood that has been shed;
there is joy for all the members
in the sorrows of the Head.

For the love of God is broader
than the measure of man's mind;
and the heart of the Eternal

is most wonderfully kind.
If our love were but more faithful,
we should take him at his word;
and our life would be thanksgiving
for the goodness of the Lord.
                                    —Frederick William Faber

Have I suffered because of my illness? Yes. Has it been frightening to go through this experience? Of course. I have had to call out for the mercy of God many times during the last few years. When my wife and I split up, I had to lean on His mercy. When I was diagnosed with a brain tumor, I had to cry out for His mercy. Without His mercy, I probably would have drunk myself to death. I have and continue to cry out for God's mercy to be shown my children.

And has God been merciful? Did He hear my cries? Did He respond to my call? If you've read my story, you know that He has. God brought me through the radiation and chemotherapy with minimal side effects and pain. He restored the paralysis on my left side. Will God be merciful to you? Absolutely! Just call on Him. He's nearby. *But you, O LORD, be not far off; O my Strength, come quickly to help me* (Psalm 22:19).

Some folks think they have to tough out life's experiences on their own. They may even reason that they got themselves into their present situation. But Psalm 22:24 states, *For he has not despised or disdained the suffering of the afflicted one; he has not hidden his face from him but has listened to his cry for help.* It is such a comfort to know that I can cry out to God for mercy whenever I need it. It's a comfort to know that nothing can happen to me that is not from God. Zechariah said, *whoever touches you, touches the apple of his eye* (Zechariah 2:8).

> *O Love that will not let me go,*
> *I rest my weary soul in Thee;*
> *I give Thee back the life I owe,*
> *That in Thine ocean depths its flow*
> *May richer, fuller be.*
>
> *O Light that followest all my way,*
> *I yield my flickering torch to Thee;*
> *My heart restores its borrowed ray,*
> *That in Thy sunshine's blaze its day*
> *May brighter, fairer be.*
>
> *O Joy that seekest me through pain,*
> *I cannot close my heart to Thee;*
> *I trace the rainbow through the rain.*
> *And feel the promise is not vain*
> *That morn shall tearless be.*
>
> *O Cross that liftest up my head,*
> *I dare not ask to fly from Thee;*
> *I lay in dust life's glory dead,*
> *And from the ground there blossoms red,*
> *Life that shall endless be.*

—George Matheson

Sometimes, all of our plans go astray and leave us feeling hopeless about the future. Our circumstances leave us broken and wounded, and we wonder how we will ever go on with our lives. Temptations assail us as the enemy comes in like a flood. But when this occurs, we need to realize that God has allowed these situations to happen and that He is with us. He will use whatever He has allowed to enter into our lives to draw us closer to Him.

God let Satan beat me down. He led me to a place in which I had to realize that He was the only One I needed. Today, I know that if I have any strength, it comes from God. I know that He gave me the power to survive. The Bible tells us that God won't give us the battle without giving us the strength. I'm *not* fond of the idea of dying, but I'm not afraid of it either.

God tested my faith to strengthen it. Through the adversity I have faced, I know today that the worse the situation, the more I should expect Him to work a miracle. In fact, the more I depend on it! I now know that I have somewhere to go with my problems, big or small. God put this tumor as my "thorn in my side" as a reminder that I will always need to depend on Him. And I do!

I no longer ask, "Why me?" I believe that God had a purpose in allowing me to have a brain tumor. So don't feel sorry for me. I'm not sorry it happened; in fact, I'm glad it did. It gave my life purpose! I have traded 30 years of quantity for six years of quality time trusting in the Lord and leaning on His mercy. Furthermore, when you look at the big picture, what have I really given up? God has promised to give me eternal life. And there is nothing on this earth that is worth giving up for eternal life.

> As life goes on
> The only words I *want* to hear
> Are, "well done, indeed."
>
> The words I *long* to hear
> Are, "well done, indeed."
>
> The words I *need* to hear
> Are, "well done, indeed,
> My good and faithful servant."

When you go through times of trials, rejoice with the apostle Peter, who said, "Praise be to the God and Father of our Lord Jesus Christ! In his great mercy he has given us new birth into a living hope through the resurrection of Jesus Christ from the dead.... In this you greatly rejoice, though now for a little while you may have had to suffer grief in all kinds of trials. These have come so that your faith—of greater worth than gold, which perishes even though refined by fire—may be proved genuine and may result in praise, glory and honor when Jesus Christ is revealed" (1 Peter 1:3,6-7).

GOD'S PROMISES

*I am in deep distress. Let us fall into the hands of the
LORD, for his mercy is great; but do not let me fall into the
hands of men.*

—2 Samuel 24:14

*Yet give attention to your servant's prayer and his plea for
mercy, O LORD my God. Hear the cry and the prayer that
your servant is praying in your presence this day.*

—1 Kings 8:28

*Forgive your people, who have sinned against you; forgive
all the offenses they have committed against you, and cause
their conquerors to show them mercy.*

—1 Kings 8:50

*Yet give attention to your servant's prayer and his plea for
mercy, O LORD my God. Hear the cry and the prayer that
your servant is praying in your presence.*

—2 Chronicles 6:19

*But in your great mercy you did not put an end to them or
abandon them, for you are a gracious and merciful.*

—Nehemiah 9:31

*Hear my cry for mercy as I call to you for help, as I lift
up my hands toward your Most Holy Place.*

—Psalm 28:2

In my alarm I said, "I am cut off from your sight!" Yet you heard my cry for mercy when I called to you for help.
—Psalm 31:22

I said, "O Lord, have mercy on me; heal me, for I have sinned against you."
—Psalm 41:4

Turn to me and have mercy on me; grant your strength to your servant and save the son of your maidservant.
—Psalm 86:16

His mercy extends to those who fear him, from generation to generation.
—Luke 1:50

Keep yourselves in God's love as you wait for the mercy of our Lord Jesus Christ to bring you to eternal life.
—Jude 1:21

Here is a trustworthy saying that deserves full acceptance: Christ Jesus came into the world to save sinners—of whom I am the worst.
But for that very reason I was shown mercy so that in me, the worst of sinners, Christ Jesus might display his unlimited patience as an example for those who would believe on him and receive eternal life.
—1 Timothy 1:15-16

…and that you, O Lord, are loving. Surely you will reward each person according to what he has done.

—Psalm 62:12

Chapter 10

IT ALL COMES
DOWN TO FAITH

I tell you the truth, if you have faith as small as a mustard seed, you can say to this mountain, "Move from here to there" and it will move. Nothing will be impossible for you.

—Matthew 17:20

George Müller was one of the great heroes of faith. An evangelist and founder of orphanages in Bristol, England, Müller cared for more than 100,000 orphans during his lifetime. Müller and his wife began working with orphans in 1836 when they prepared their own home in Bristol to accommodate 30 girls. Soon after the establishment of this first home, three more houses were furnished, and the total of children cared for grew to 130.

In 1845, as growth continued, Müller decided that a separate building needed to be designed to house 300 additional children. In 1849, at Ashley Down, Bristol,

Müller opened that home. By 1870, more than 2,000 children were being accommodated in five homes.

A story is told that Müller's orphan children once had all eaten their dinners and went happily off to bed. However, what the unsuspecting orphans did not know was that the orphanage had no money for their breakfasts the next day. Although Müller did not know how God would provide, he was confident the Lord would come through for the children. After all, he reasoned, wasn't God a father to the fatherless (see Psalm 68:5)?

Müller went to bed, in faith committing the care of the orphans to God. The next morning, as he went for a walk, he prayed for God to supply the children's needs. While walking, Müller met a friend who asked him to accept some money for the orphanage. Müller thanked him and then went back to the orphanage for breakfast.

Müller never once made a request for financial support. He did not take a salary, nor did he go into debt, even though the five homes cost a total of more than £100,000 to build. Many times, he received unsolicited food donations only hours before they were needed to feed the children, further strengthening his faith in God. Müller claimed that during his lifetime, 50,000 of his specific prayers were answered—5,000 of which his diary confirmed were answered on the same day he prayed them. "I live in the spirit of prayer," he said. "I pray as I walk about, when I lie down, and when I rise up. And the answers are always coming. When once I am persuaded that a thing is right and for the glory of God, I go on praying for it until the answer comes. George Müller never gives up!"

Müller's faith extended beyond the realm of finances. In August of 1877, he and his wife boarded a boat in Bristol, England, to head to North America. Off the coast of Newfoundland, the weather turned cold and the ship's progress was seriously slowed by fog. The captain had been on the bridge for 24 hours. Then something happened that would change his life.

Müller appeared on the bridge and said, "Captain, I've come to tell you I must be in Quebec by Saturday afternoon."

"It's impossible," said the captain.

"Very well," said Müller, "if your ship cannot take me, God will find some other way. I have never broken an engagement for 52 years. Let us go down to the chart room and pray."

The Captain wondered which lunatic asylum Müller had escaped from. "Mr. Müller," he said, "do you know how dense this fog is?"

"No," replied Müller. "My eyes are not on the density of the fog, but on the living God, who controls every circumstance of my life." Müller then knelt down and prayed. When he had finished, the captain was about to pray, but Müller put his hand on his shoulder and gave him two reasons not to do so.

"First, you do not believe God will provide," he said. "Second, I believe He has, and there is no need whatever for you to pray about it." The captain looked at Müller in amazement.

"Captain," Müller continued, "I have known my Lord for 52 years, and there has never been a single day that I have failed to get an audience with the King. Get up, sir, and open the door. You will find that the fog is gone." The captain walked to the door and opened it. The fog had lifted. It was the captain who later told the story of this incident, and he was later described by a well-known evangelist as "one of the most devoted men I ever knew."

Müller loved to say, "Work with all your might; but trust not in the least in your work." His faith that his prayers for finances would be answered was rooted in his belief in the sovereignty of God. He would often say, "*How* the means are to come, I know not; but I know that God is almighty, that the hearts of all are in His hands, and that, if He pleases to influence persons, they will send help." His aim in life was to glorify God by helping people take God at His word. In order to fully understand the concept of faith and trust, he saturated his soul with the Word of God.

By the time Müller died, he had read the Bible through 200 times. His aim was to see God in Jesus Christ crucified and raised from the dead, thereby maintaining the happiness of his soul in God. By this deep satisfaction in God, George Mueller was set free from fear and disbelief.

The only thing God does not own, and the thing He wants
most from you, is the praise of your heart.
—Charles Stanley

We have only to look at the great "faith chapter" of
the Bible in Hebrews 11 to see that God takes care of
those who put their trust in Him. Let's look at the roster
of those who lived by faith that this chapter in Hebrews
provides.

By faith, Abel offered to God a more pleasing sacrifice
than did Cain. By faith, Enoch vanished from earth into
the presence of God without experiencing death. By faith,
Noah built an ark to save his family.

By faith, Abraham traveled to a place he had never
been, even though he did not know where he was going.
By faith, even though he was old and his wife, Sarah, was
barren, he trusted in God's promise that he would have
descendents like the stars of the heaven. And because he
had faith and believed God was faithful and that His promises were valid, he became the father of a great nation.

By faith, Abraham offered Isaac as a sacrifice when God
commanded him to do so. By faith, Isaac blessed Jacob
and Esau in regard to their future. By faith, Jacob, when
he was dying, blessed each of Joseph's sons and worshiped
as he leaned on the top of his staff.

By faith, Joseph, when his end was near, spoke about
the Exodus of the Israelites from Egypt. By faith, Moses'
parents were not afraid to defy Pharaoh's edict to kill
every newborn child and hid Moses for three months

after he was born. By faith, Moses, when he had grown up, refused to be known as the son of Pharaoh's daughter. By faith, he did not fear the king's anger, left Egypt, and persevered because he saw Him who is invisible. By faith, he kept the Passover and the sprinkling of blood, so that the destroyer of the firstborn would not touch the firstborn of Israel.

By faith, the Children of Israel passed through the Red Sea as on dry land. Later, when they reached the Promised Land, by faith, they marched around the walls of Jericho, which fell down before them. By faith, the prostitute Rahab, because she welcomed the spies, was not killed with those who were disobedient.

By faith, Gideon fought the enemy with a handful of soldiers and some lamps. By faith, Samson pushed the pillars of the temple, bringing the roof crashing down on the enemy. By faith, David slew the giant Goliath. By faith, Daniel survived the lion's den. By faith, many more heroes stayed true to God's calling right up to the present day.

That brings us to my story. When I became so desperately ill, I was like Peter. When Jesus asked the disciples if they would abandon Him like so many others had, Peter responded, *"Lord, to whom shall we go? You have the words of eternal life. We believe and know that you are the Holy One of God"* (John 6:68-69). I too had no one to go to and nowhere to turn but to God. And isn't that the best place to be anyway, safe in the arms of Jesus?

There are good ideas, and then there are God's ideas.

It's human nature to not want to serve a master. The concept of a God who created us to serve Him and who would in turn take care of our needs if we have faith in Him is alien to us. From the moment we are conceived, we are taught to depend on someone else. We then come to believe that our greatest accomplishment is in attaining independence. But many times, independence breeds pride. Even little children say, "I do it myself." And as we grow, we learn more and more to depend on ourselves. We say, "Look what I did all on my own!"

This desire to be in control of our situation—our own life—has been around for a long time. That's what happened to Adam and Eve in the Garden. They thought they knew better than God. They stopped trusting Him. They took their lives into their own hands. And they lost everything.

The hardest thing to do is to have faith in God and let Him take care of our problems and needs. Faith and obedience cannot be separated. Obedience to God is a direct result of true faith in Him. The great evangelist Spurgeon said, "Faith and obedience are bound up in the same bundle. He that obeys God, trusts God; and he that trusts God obeys God."

Faith and worry also cannot coexist. Trusting God and having faith means that we stop worrying and trust Him completely for all our needs, both physically and spiritually. Jeremy Taylor once said, "It is impossible for that man to despair who remembers that his Helper is omnipotent." H.W. Shaw adds, "Faith is the soul riding at anchor."

Trying to live our lives without faith in God is like watching a parade from ground level while God watches from a rooftop. He can already see the beginning and the end. He knows what will happen. He is in control. He makes the impossible possible.

Isn't it comforting to know that you have a Source that you can turn to for any issue you are facing? Isn't it comforting to know that God can take any problem and turn it into the best resolution possible? Isn't it comforting to realize that God knows the best way for things to work out in your life so that you don't have to worry about it? That's peace!

One of the most "godly" things we can do is slow down.
—Joyce Meyer

As I look back on my situation, I realize that a great deal of good has come out of my being diagnosed with an inoperable brain tumor. Now, I wake up to life each day. I appreciate everything about my life, but especially my family and friends. I have learned a great deal of humility in a short amount of time, which is timely because the idea that there is a God who watches over me has become a tangible reality in my life. I have a new amazement for the nature of God, especially when I consider that the same mighty God who could create the world through the power of His voice could also reach down and hold a baby in His arms.

I now realize that the purpose of this life may in fact be to experience life, to learn hard lessons about the battles between good and evil, and to forever learn to have faith in God. Above all, because of my experience, I can now honestly agree with James when he writes, *Consider it pure joy, my brothers, whenever you face trials of many kinds, because you know that the testing of your faith develops perseverance. Perseverance must finish its work so that you may be mature and complete, not lacking anything* (James 1:2-4).

Without a doubt, you will face difficult challenges during your life. When these times come your way, you need to keep your chin up and come out swinging. Remember that God has brought this situation into your life to refine you with His fire and bring you closer to Himself. Also remember that others are watching to see how you will handle your challenges. If you keep fighting, people will admire your spirit, your courage, your strength, and your stamina.

Good luck to you! May God bless everyone!

I've never made a fortune
and it's probably too late now.
But I don't worry about that much,
I'm happy anyhow.

And as I go along life's way,
I'm reaping better than I sowed.
I'm drinking from my saucer,
'Cause my cup has overflowed.

I don't have a lot of riches,
and sometimes the going's tough.
But I've got loved ones around me,
and that makes me rich enough.

I thank God for his blessings,
and the mercies He's bestowed.
I'm drinking from my saucer,
'Cause my cup has overflowed.

I remember times when things went wrong,
My faith wore somewhat thin.
But all at once the dark clouds broke,
and the sun peeped through again.

So God, help me not to gripe about
the tough rows that I've hoed.
I'm drinking from my saucer,
'Cause my cup has overflowed.

If God gives me strength and courage,
when the way grows steep and rough.
I'll not ask for other blessings,
I'm already blessed enough.

And may I never be too busy,
to help others bear their loads.
Then I'll keep drinking from my saucer,
'Cause my cup has overflowed.

—Anonymous

GOD'S PROMISES

He replied, "You of little faith, why are you so afraid?" Then he got up and rebuked the winds and the waves, and it was completely calm.

—Matthew 8:26

But Jesus turned around, and when He saw her He said, "Be of good cheer, daughter; your faith has made you well." And the woman was made well from that hour.

—Matthew 9:22 NKJV

This righteousness from God comes through faith in Jesus Christ to all who believe.

—Romans 3:22

Therefore, since we have been justified through faith, we have peace with God through our Lord Jesus Christ.

—Romans 5:21

So then faith comes by hearing, and hearing by the word of God.

—Romans 10:17 NKJV

POSTSCRIPT

William Barclay relates the following story: Three apprentice devils were coming to Earth to finish their apprenticeship. They were talking to Satan, the chief of devils, about their plans to tempt and to ruin men.

The first said, "I will tell them that there is no God."

Satan said, "That will not delude many, for they know that there is a God."

The second said, "I will tell men there is no hell."

Satan answered, "You will deceive no one that way; men know even now that there is a hell for sin."

The third said, "I will tell men that there is no hurry."

"Go," said Satan, "and you will ruin men by the thousands. The most dangerous of all delusions is that there is plenty of time."

John 3:16 states, *For God so loved the world that he gave his one and only Son, that whoever believes in him shall not perish but have eternal life.* God loves you. He created you. He would do anything for you if you would just surrender your life to Him.

If you have never asked God to be Lord of your life, I urge you to do it now. How? The following Scriptures will provide you with a clear path to salvation.

1. Believe That You Are a Sinner

As it is written: "There is no one righteous, not even one"

—Romans 3:10).

For all have sinned and fall short of the glory of God .
—Romans 3:23

2. Realize That You Can't "Earn" Salvation

For it is by grace you have been saved, through faith—and this not from yourselves, it is the gift of God—not by works, so that no one can boast.

—Ephesians 2:8-9

But someone will say, "You have faith; I have deeds." Show me your faith without deeds, and I will show you my faith by what I do.

—James 2:18

3. Believe That God Has Provided for Your Sin

For the wages of sin is death, but the gift of God is eternal life in Christ Jesus our Lord.

—Romans 6:23

But God demonstrates his own love for us in this: While we were still sinners, Christ died for us.

—Romans 5:8

4. Believe That if You Confess Your Sins, God Will Forgive You

If you confess with your mouth, "Jesus is Lord," and believe in your heart that God raised him from the dead, you will be saved. For it is with your heart that you believe and are justified, and it is with your mouth that you confess and are saved.

—Romans 10:9-10

Everyone who calls on the name of the Lord will be saved.

—Romans 10:13

Christ died for sins once for all, the righteous for the unrighteous, to bring you to God. He was put to death in the body but made alive by the Spirit.

—1 Peter 3:18

5. Invite God into Your Life!

If you want to accept Christ as your Savior, say the following prayer:

Dear Lord Jesus,
I admit that I am a sinner. Your Word clearly shows me that fact.
I know that Jesus Christ died to take away my sin.

Now, dear Lord, please forgive me all my sins
and make me Your child.
In Jesus' name I pray, amen.

You have just prayed to God, confessing that you're a sinner and telling Him that you believe Jesus died for your sins on the cross. You have asked Him to come into your heart and life. Now tell Him you love Him and that you want to live with Him forever in Heaven. When you have done these things, you will have become a child of God for eternity.

RECOMMENDED BOOKS

Our Daily Bread (Daily Devotional)
  RBC Press

Traveling Light
  Max Lucado

It's Not About Me
  Max Lucado

Tempered Steel
  Steve Farrar

King Me
  Steve Farrar

Wild at Heart
  John Eldredge

Six Battles Every Man Must Win
  Bill Perkins

The Purpose Driven Life
  Rick Warren"

A Bend in the Road
  David Jeremiah

The Prayer of Jabez
  Bruce Wilkinson

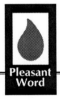

CPSIA information can be obtained at www.ICGtesting.com
Printed in the USA
BVOW071329220812

298487BV00002B/3/A